The 7-Day Herbal Tea

Lung Detox

Cleanse, Heal, and Strengthen Your Lungs
With The Power Of Healing Herbal Tea

Josh Williams

www.LivingHerbalTea.com

First Edition 2013
ISBN-13: 978-1489542960
ISBN-10: 1489542965

Table Of Contents

Introduction - 01

The Lungs - 03

The Power Of Breath - 08

Herbal Tea Essentials – 14

The Lung Detox Herbs - 24

The 7-Day Lung Detox - 36

Empowering Lung Exercises - 40

Lung Loving Herbal Tea Recipes - 46

References - 52

About The Author - 53

INTRODUCTION

I smoked cigarettes for over 15 years, and I started while my body was still growing. I cannot even begin to imagine the damage I did to my respiratory and cardiovascular systems during those years, but I can imagine how much worse it could have been without he healing power of plant medicine. I relied on herbal tea during my quit and over the years since and I honestly believe that my success and my health have depended on it.

One thing is for sure - you don't have to be an ex-smoker like me to give extra love to your lungs. Like your heart, your lungs work all day every day providing a service that you literally could not live without. There are many factors that can take away from how well our lungs perform, and if these factors are part of your life, a lung detox may be just the thing you need. Some of the things that get in the way of optimal lung health include...

- Smoking now or in the past
- Living in a polluted environment
- Spending a great deal of time indoors
- Leading a sedentary lifestyle
- Being surrounded by environmental irritants
- Dealing with recurring allergies or other respiratory complaints
- Improper or shallow breathing habits

How many of us don't check off at least one of those things? The good news is that a simple, extremely inexpensive, and truly enjoyable herbal tea lung detox has

1

the power to help your lungs in some amazing ways. The herbal teas we'll be exploring in this book can help…

- Clear out phlegm and mucous
- Soothe smooth muscle lining within the lungs
- Cleanse toxins
- Create healthy new mucous linings
- Remove blockages and phlegm plugs
- Increase lung circulation
- Deepen and relax breathing
- Stop inflammation cycles
- Heal lung imbalances
- Nourish the lungs with essential vitamins and minerals

Pretty amazing, right?

In this book I am going to introduce you to a nearly effortless 7-day program that will bathe your lungs in the healing power of four beautiful herbs known for their relationship to one of our most precious body systems. These herbs are easy to find, simple to prepare, and a treat to sip each day. As we go on I'll teach you how to select the herbs, how to brew the perfect healing herbal tea, how to experience the most gentle and effective lung detox possible, and I'll even introduce you to some important ideas about breathing and exercising your lungs.

Take a deep breath and turn the page to get started!

THE LUNGS

In this section I'd like to give you a really brief look at just how amazing our lungs are. Understanding what's happening in your chest when you breathe can help create a deeper relationship with your lungs and deeper level of gratitude and respect. The more we know about how our body works optimally, the more aware we are when something isn't going right. Don't worry; this won't be a complicated anatomy and physiology lesson with homework. I just want to shed a little light on the amazing respiratory system before we move on.

The Air We Breathe

The lungs work all the time. From slow and steady breathing while we sleep to heavy breathing while we exercise, the lungs are always working hard to give our bodies the fuel and nourishment they need to succeed.

The core function of the lungs is to expel carbon dioxide – a byproduct of body functions, and draw in oxygen which fuels many of the things our body does. The lungs bring in oxygen on the inhalation and send out carbon dioxide when we exhale. A pretty smooth operation!

When we breathe properly, the diaphragm muscle which is located at the base of the rib cage, and the intercostals muscles which are in between all of our ribs open up the chest cavity to that air is drawn in. Many people think that we force air into our lungs, but we actually gently draw it in by enlarging the chest cavity like a bellows.

When air reaches the depths of the lungs it ends up in the alveoli. Alveolus are tiny air sacs with very thin walls. The oxygen within the air gets passed through these walls to oxygen-carrying red blood cells at the same time that those cells pass off the carbon dioxide to be released on the next exhalation. That's a whole lot of action taking place in one breath. Let's break it down to make sure it all sinks in…

At the inhalation…

Air is drawn into the lungs via a muscle contraction. The air passes down into the bronchioles of the lungs until it ends up in countless tiny air sacs. Once in the sacs, the oxygen within the air is passed through to a red blood cell that is carrying carbon dioxide. A switch takes place as the oxygen boards the red blood cell via binding to the hemoglobin in the red blood cell and the previously held carbon dioxide is passed through the air sac wall into the lungs.

At the exhalation…

The muscles of the rib cage and diaphragm expand to push the carbon dioxide content of the lungs out into the air. Once we are free from the used gasses in the lungs, the signal is sent to inhale a fresh breath of oxygen-rich air!

Imagine all of that taking place in the course of one breath. Consider also the many signals, chemical changes, pH changes, and other actions happening to let the body know when to breath, how fast to breathe, and what to do with the breath once it comes in. It's all pretty amazing.

Strong And Sensitive

The lungs are made from a spongy tissue that is able to easily expand, contract, and stretch as we breathe. This tissue has to be tough in order to maintain its shape and power over our entire lifetime. Think about it – the lungs work 24 hours a day, 7 days a week. That's a lot more time than any body builder could spend working any single muscle group! That being said, the lungs are extremely sensitive. They are usually the first responders when it comes to allergies, air born viruses, and many illnesses. We're breathing all the time so it makes sense that our lungs see a good deal of the things that challenge our health.

The reason why we don't get sick every single time we inhale a mouthful of exhaust, the floating remnants of someone's sneeze, or mold in the air is because of mucous. This gooey substance lines the walls of the lungs and acts like a trap to anything that shouldn't be in there while also keeping the entire respiratory system protected and hydrated. In order for air to get into the deepest parts of the lungs where the air sacs are, they pass through channel after channel of mucous lined airways that get increasing smaller as they go giving the lungs as many chances as possible to catch foreign debris, bacteria, mold, viruses, and allergens.

Mucous is usually expelled from the body via sneezing, coughing, or being assimilated once it's full of gunk. If we have healthy lung function this is no problem, but most of us can use a little help to do some deep lung cleaning once or twice a year.

Common Troublemakers

As strong as the respiratory system is, there are many things that can prevent it from performing optimally. Some of the issues that can prevent the lungs from working, cleansing, and balancing properly include...

- Respiratory diseases like asthma, COPD, and emphysema
- Recurring respiratory infections
- Poor breathing habits
- Allergies
- Pollution
- Irritants
- Chemicals
- Poor diet
- Dehydration

These issues cause individual people trouble in varying ways, but the good news is that we can help the lungs along through detox protocols, learning to breathe properly, and through helping to create world where all of the air we breathe is clean and safe. As we move on we'll be exploring a gentle and effective 7-day lung detox that is both simple and affordable. If you have a respiratory illness or difficulty breathing, I strongly encourage you to see a doctor before embarking on any kind of respiratory healing program – even a natural one. Herbs, teas, exercises, and diets can all be extremely effective in helping heal the lungs, but it's all best done with the guidance of your primary healthcare giver.

Clean and Clear

As we move on we're going to explore a little but more about the lungs and the function of breathing. I want to cover this topic because I think the ways in which healthy breathing affects our lives is absolutely stunning. Proper breathing can influence everything from mood and migraines to immunity and weight loss. Sounds pretty important, right?

Once we get acquainted with the importance of healthy breathing, we'll start the tea party and look at simple ways to make healing herbal tea in your own kitchen, which herbs to use, and how to complete a 7-day lung detox the easy way.

THE POWER OF BREATH

As we explored in the previous chapter, breathing is an essential part of fueling and cleansing the body – but it doesn't stop there. Our breath plays an integral role in our moods, ability to deal with stress, immune response, our digestion, the health of our visceral organs, digestion, and a whole lot more. Who knew?

In order to benefit from all of the amazing things that breathing can do for our health we have to breathe in a healthy way on two levels. First, we have to be able to breathe. This means clear lungs with healthy mucous linings, no inflammation, and healthy function. Second, we have to breathe correctly. Most of us are trained to suck in our stomachs and breathe with the muscles in our shoulders and chest which is the opposite of how it should be done.

When the lungs are healthy and clean we are able to take in more air without forcing or straining. The oxygen in the air we inhale is more readily absorbed into our bodies, and the carbon dioxide waste makes it way out of our bodies in a more effective way. The less healthy the lungs are, the weaker their performance.

When we breathe properly we use the right muscles and get air into the deepest parts of the lungs where the most effective respiration takes place. When we breathe using our diaphragm, our organs get a gentle detoxifying massage with each breathe and our digestion is supported. Proper breathing creates a sense of well-being in the body since it is slow, deep, and steady, so it cuts back drastically on stress and anxiety which means that we feel calmer, clearer, and less reactive. Proper breathing also supports the immune system by keeping us out of stress cycles and cutting down on how many of our resources get used in the wrong ways.

The 7-day lung detox is all about helping nourish your lungs with essential vitamins and minerals that are believed to help them heal and be strong. It also works by cleansing, clearing, and soothing them. You'll be letting the herbal tea do a great deal of the work during the detox, but it's important that if you aren't breathing properly to begin with that you work on it. I'll give you some simple exercises later on in the book that will help you gently train your body and mind back into a state of effortless, healing breath cycles.

In order to find out just how healthy your breathing is, let's do a simple exercise. Find a comfortable space where you feel like you can relax and let go. You can stand or sit, but make sure that your back is straight either way. Follow the steps below one at a time, and go at a pace that feels right for you. If you get too uncomfortable at any point, end the exercise and come back later on.

- Allow your body and mind to relax. Don't force it. Just get centered and comfortable where you are and choose to be present in this moment.
- Bring your attention to your mouth and nose. Take note of where you inhale and where you exhale.

Do you breathe with your nose, your mouth, or a combination of the two?

- Try to feel the breathe coming into your body at the point of your mouth or nose. Just experience the small sensations created there with each inhalation and exhalation.
- Now, follow your breath when you inhale and try to feel it enter into your body. Do the same by feeling it leave your body when you exhale.
- What parts of your body move, contract, flex, relax, or open up when you breathe? Spend as much time as you need to really take inventory about what your whole body does when you inhale and when you exhale. Try to remember what happens.
- Now, go ahead and take a really slow and deep breath. Try to breathe as deeply as you possibly can. While you do this, pay close attention to which muscles and areas of your body move, flex, and stretch.
- Once you have a good idea of how your body responds to breathing, gently let your breath return to normal and end this exercise.

For many people this will be the first time they've gotten in touch with all of the little movements and adjustments the body makes in order to breathe. It's all pretty interesting, right?

Now that you've successfully completed this exercise, you can learn a lot about how healthy your breathing is. Let's explore.

Unhealthy Breathing

If you noticed that your shoulders, shoulder blades, upper chest, pectoral muscles, sides, or upper arms moved, flexed, or adjusted as you breathed, you are probably not breathing as well as you could. If your belly stays held in or does not expand on an inhalation, you may be holding your breathing muscles in for fear of looking like you have a big belly – this is torture on your respiratory system! Similarly, if you notice that you inhale primarily through your mouth, or that your mouth tends to be open when you inhale through your nose, your breathing is not what it could be.

Some of the reasons that we learn to breathe poorly include sitting too long, trying to hold our bellies in to appear thin, forcing an unnatural posture, being afraid of making sound when we breathe, worrying about sending our breath out into the world, subtle subconscious fears about receiving the air around us, and so on. Babies are born breathing beautifully – we learn how to do it wrong over time, usually in our teenage years.

Never fear! Learning the right way that gives all of the amazing benefits I shared earlier is a really easy process and I'll walk you through it later on in the book.

Healthy Breathing

A healthy breath happens in the belly, just under the navel. The diaphragm muscle which attaches below the rib cage is pulled down into the gut on an inhalation. This movement gently draws the breath into the lungs while the

11

belly expands as the organs are massaged. The upper body is almost completely still except for some gentle expansion in the chest to make room for the fresh air.

Inhalation should take place exclusively through the nose. The mouth and throat are not equipped to catch foreign particles in the air, add humidity to the breath, or regulate its temperature. Mouth breathing causes unfiltered air that is usually dried out and the wrong temperature to rush into the lungs too quickly. Nasal breathing gives your body plenty of time and space to cleanse and regulate the air so that it doesn't bring in germs, dry you out, or cause damage to the delicate lung linings. Remember, the lungs are lined with mucous partly to keep them moist and hydrated – dry mouth breathing works against what your body is trying so hard to accomplish.

If your breathing is not great, or if you go between good breathing and poor breathing, you've come to the right place. We're going to get back on track with gentle, healthy, healing breathing as part of the 7-day lung detox and you can expect to have your life changed because of this. Breathing may seem simple, but when it's done poorly it causes a whole host of issues that you simply don't have to suffer through.

From calming and immune strength to better metabolic function and digestion, proper breathing is an essential in having healthy lungs, a healthy body, and a healthy mind. It's no coincidence that the world's many meditation and contemplative traditions all spend so much time on learning to breathe properly.

In the next chapter I'm going to give you the essential basics to working with herbal tea. I'll tell you all about why herbal tea is such an amazing healing force, how to select the best herbs for any tea you want to enjoy, how to brew the perfect cup every time, and how much tea you should drink to get great benefits. After that, we'll explore the four amazing herbs that make up the 7-day lung detox program and I'll tell you how they work, what they'll do for you, and how to work with them. By the end of the next two chapters you'll know everything you need to know to get your inexpensive herbs, any brewing gear you may not already have on hand, and get to enjoying the gentle healing benefits of medicinal herbal tea!

HERBAL TEA ESSENTIALS

In this chapter I'm going to arm you with all the information you need to create amazing herbal tea brews each and every time – no matter which healing plants you happen to work with. Herbal tea is a poplar healing option because of how easy it is to use and how much it engages us consciously in the process of working with it. By the end of this section you'll be ready to create amazing herbal tea like a pro!

What Is Herbal Tea?

Herbal tea is created by steeping parts of plants in either hot or cold water in order to infuse the water with the healing properties of that plant. Leaves, flowers, stems, roots, rhizomes, and even bark all show up in the herbal tea world depending on what plant is being used and which part of is it beneficial in healing.

In most cases herbal tea is made using dried herbs. When a plant is dried the cell walls break down and the nutrients, minerals, vitamins, and essential oils become more available. Many plants also lose toxicity after being dried, so this can be a safer method as well. Fresh herbs can certainly be used in herbal tea, but you should consult a professional before doing so.

When dried herbs are soaked in hot or cold water, they spring back to life and their inner goodness is merged with the water itself. Steeping herbs in hot water is the classic way to prepare herbal tea, but you can make equally effective herbal tea via a cold soak method. We'll cover both in detail later on.

For now, just remember that herbal tea is any drink made my infusing water with the healing properties of various plants and their various parts.

How Herbal Tea Works

Plants are simply amazing. They each carry a unique array of healing profiles that range from simple vitamins and minerals to complex chemical combinations that help create positive change when taken.

Herbal tea delivers the healing properties of herbs into the body in a truly absorbable and friendly way. Water is essential to the human body and when it is saturated with healing qualities, the body is better able to absorb and use it. When tea is sipped, the entire natural digestion process starting with the sense of smell and the lips gets involved in the process. I believe that pills are less effective because they are tasteless and often odorless. A pill doesn't give the body any time to process, greet, and approve a remedy. Tea, on the other hand, bathes the tongue and other senses which can help the body relax and let its defenses down.

When working with herbal tea we are working with the same essential principles that govern all herbal and nutritional medicine. We open ourselves up to the specific healing abilities of various plants to create positive support, change, and transformation within the body, mind, emotions, and energy systems.

Selecting Herbs

One of the most important things to consider when using healing herbal tea is which herbs to actually make your tea from. There are thousands of herbs, so it can seem overwhelming to know which ones are best. Books on the subject of herbal remedies are a great way to start, and books like this one that speak specifically about herbal tea are even better if you prefer tea to other herbal delivery methods.

Before selecting any herbs to use in tea, look at them from a general healing level, then from the level of use in herbal tea. If you can't find any information about them from tea experts, it's probably for a reason. Not all medicinal herbs translate well to herbal tea blends, but most do.

Another thing to consider is how to buy your herbs. Picking up pre-packaged tea bags is simple, but may not be as good for you. In order for herbs to be placed in bas they have to be pulverized which increases their surface area and causes them to break down and lose healing potency very fast. Packaged tea bags are also rarely marked with packaging dates so you never really know how long the tea has been in there. I also don't favor herbs in this format because they have been handled so much and have been taken far from their original form. That being said, if pre-packaged herbal tea is all you can work with or access – by all means go for it! My preference, and that of most herbal tea enthusiasts, is whole herbs. You can buy these from shops online and in person, and they are surprisingly easy and fun to work with. Whole herbs maintain the color, aroma, and texture that the plant was meant to have, and they give you the chance to create a deeper and more intimate bond with the plant before you drink it. I buy all of my bulk herbs online at really low prices and store them away until needed. I have figured out that I save a great deal of money buying whole herbs over high-end organic pre-packaged options, so that's something to consider as well.

Storing Your Herbs

If you buy tea bags, keep them in their package as much as you can. You may also consider buying a small light and air proof container, or choosing a cool drawer, to store your tea collection in. This will help prevent the tea from weakening too quickly. Light, heat, and air all break down herbs – so do what you can to keep your herbs free from these elements.

If you purchase whole or bulk herbs, you need to be extra careful about storage. The company I buy from sells handy 4 and 8 ounce bags that seal tight. I keep my herbs in the bags they come in because the quality is right. All of my herb bags live in large opaque sweater boxes that I keep stacked nicely in the coolest part of my kitchen; an area free from any direct heat or sunlight. You could also store your whole herbs in colored glass jars, canning jars stored in a dark place, or in special herb storage bins. I lean towards the frugal, so I find it best to just buy herbs that already come in great packaging that won't go straight to the landfill.

Longevity

Most tea bags are good for about a year. Bulk herbs that have been well cared for can last for several years. Many herbal healing enthusiasts will put a one year time limit on any whole herbs they keep, but I favor letting the plant tell me when it's time to be composted. When the color, smell, taste, or texture of the herbs starts to take a turn, it's time to put the remainder of the herbs into a compost pile, in a wild place, or in a garden. If you ever see mold, mildew, traces of water, foul smells, or other alarming things, get rid of your herbs immediately and work on identifying what cause the issue.

Basic Brewing Gear

In order to make a great cup of healing herbal tea, there are a few things you'll need to have on hand. This list reflects the basics, but you're welcome to add on anything else you think is important...

- Tea kettle or dedicated water-only sauce pan
- Heat-proof tea mug
- Infuser
- Your herbs or pre-packaged tea bags
- A tea towel

Your tea kettle should be made for boiling water. Some tea kettles are decorative or are meant to hold water that's already been boiled somewhere else. This is more a formal tea service type implement that doesn't have a great deal of use in making healing tea – although you are welcome to use them if you enjoy the ritual of it all. A proper kettle will be metal and usually will be lined with ceramic or enamel. These are meant to sit on a flame or heating element safely.

Mugs can be purchased just about anywhere. My favorite healing herbal tea mug is a regular old coffee mug handed down to me by my Grandmother. If you've never seen all the novelty and fanciful mugs out there – you're in for a treat!

Infusers come in an endless variety. Many people opt for the simple infuser ball or spoon. These allow you to trap your herbs inside a mesh or perforated apparatus which is submerged into your hot water. Other options include infuser pots, infuser mugs, and even infusers that drain the automatically into your mug when placed on top of it. Have fun looking at infusers since they will be the center of your tea making process.

Keep an absorbent towel on hand in case of spills. Be mindful when working with hot water because even just-boiling water can cause serious burns!

Brewing Hot Herbal Tea

The process for creating amazing hot herbal tea is really simple…

- Bring clean water to the point just before it starts to boil while you prepare your herbs or tea bag

- Pour the hot water into your mug over the tea bag or your infuser. If you're using a self-contained infuser pot or mug, pour directly into that.
- Glance at the clock so that you can brew your herbs for the right amount of time. We'll cover this in detail next.
- Take time to connect with the aroma, color, and process while it happens – this can help your body feel at ease with taking the tea.
- Remove the tea bag or infuser, or otherwise separate the herbs from the water once the time is up.
- Wait for the water to be a safe and comforting temperature, and then let the healing begin!

While there isn't a general rule that applies to all herbs as far as brewing times, most herbs will fall within a time frame you can fine tune with experience. The herbs discussed later on in the 7-day lung detox will be great with the times below.

Leaves and flowers : 6-7 minutes
Stalks and stems : 7-8 minutes
Roots and rhizomes : 8-10 minutes
Bark : 10-12 minutes, or use a concoction method

The herbs we'll talk about later on are all leaves, so a 6 minute brewing time on the average is ideal.

Brewing Cold Herbal Tea

This is a really fun way to create warm-weather healing drinks, and it's really simple. I use a lidded canning jar and it works perfectly. You can use any glass jar with a tight-fitting lid.

- Fill your jar with 6-8 ounces of cool, clean water
- Add your herbal blend or tea bags
- Secure lid
- Place in refrigerator
- Wait 4-6 hours for leaves and flowers, 5-7 hours for stems, and up to 12 hours for roots. Taste at hourly intervals to find the right brewing time for any specific blend you may work with.
- Remove tea bags or separate herbs from water using a sieve or infuser screen
- Pour tea into a big glass, add ice or cut with cold water, and enjoy!

If you want to use ice you'll need to make your tea stronger than will be discussed later on. I would add 50% more herbs to any brew when ice will be involved. If you plan on drinking your brew without ice, add a pinch more or around 10% more, since cold brewing is less intense than hot.

Sipping

The process of enjoying your healing herbal tea should be special. Don't rush it to treat it like a canned soda. After all, we're talking about your health here!

If possible, sit and enjoy your herbal tea while meditating on, visualizing, praying about, or just keeping positive thoughts about your healing goals. Choose to let each sip bring you closer and closer to the good places you want to be in your life. Consciously allow the tea to work *with* you and really try to stay connected to it. If you treat the process of enjoying your herbal tea like a type of active meditation, manifestation, or prayer, you are more likely to see the plant energies go to work for you faster. Part of this is due to things happening on what we might call the 'spiritual level', while others are on the level of simply helping your body feel safe and receptive to the work the plants are capable of doing.

Let the herbs help you follow your heart.

Dosages

Like most things herbal tea, there are no hard and fast rules here, but it is easy to stay within a safe zone.

Most hot herbal tea blends should be made using one full to heaping teaspoon *in total* per 8 ounces of water. This means that if you have 4 herbs in your blend, you'll mix and match to get one teaspoon in total. You may have ½ teaspoon of one herb and a pinch of the other three, ¼ teaspoon of each, or some other combination. Do what works for you over time. With the recipes I'll share in this book I'll give specific dosing for each to take the guesswork out of it for you. Most pre-packaged tea bags contain exactly one teaspoon or an otherwise appropriate dosage of the featured herb.

When making iced herbal tea use up to 2 teaspoons of herbs per 8 ounces of water when several ice cubes will be used. If you won't be using ice but will be brewing in the fridge, use a heaping teaspoon.

Most herbalists suggest drinking an 8 ounce herbal tea up to three times per day during an illness or imbalance. This tends to be a good amount for most people, but many herbs can be taken more regularly if needed. I suggest starting with a slowly-sipped cup early in the day and going from there. If you feel you need more, add a cup 4-6 hours later. Always take the smallest amount needed by your body. For the lung detox tea we'll be drinking twice per day throughout the 7-day program, but you can cut down to once or go up to three times if you feel it is necessary or if you've been directed to do so by an herbal or medical professional.

In the next section we'll be meeting the four specific herbs used in the 7-day lung detox, and several other herbs that have a healing relationship with the lungs and respiratory system as well. By the end of that chapter you'll be well versed about lung loving herbs that help clear, cleanse, detox, strengthen, and nourish!

THE LUNG DETOX HERBS

In the next section we'll be going over every simple step of the 7-day lung detox. A big part of those steps will include working with at least four medicinal herbs that have a very long and very well respected relationship with healing and empowering the lungs and their various functions. The four main herbs could be considered the 'best of the best' when it comes to all around lung detoxification, cleansing, and healing. I'll be including several others for your reference that you are free to try as part of the detox or later on for even more variety in nourishing and loving your lungs.

Before purchasing any of these herbs, please read their individual profiles to make sure they are right for you. If any herb doesn't look or feel right for you, or if your medical professional doesn't think you should work with it, choose something else from the list to replace it. Although the first four herbs are the best, there's no harm in replacing them if you need to. Also, please ensure that you purchase the right organic herbs by verifying their Latin names as provided.

Mullein
Verbascum thapus
Leaves and flowers

Mullein is my absolute favorite when it comes to all things lung related. This gentle herb seems to focus its energy in a very effective way in the lungs, and it gets to work fast!

Mullein helps remove any 'gunk' from with the lungs via its gentle yet thorough expectorant abilities. It helps the lungs purge themselves of mucous and phlegm that have taken their fill of toxins, pollutants, and foreign matter so that it can be given healthy replacements.

Like many herbs used in herbal tea, mullein has natural mucilage which soothes, coats, and protects the respiratory system from the mouth to the lungs.

In many cases, recurring lung issues are wrapped up in an inflammation cycle. Mullein is a gentle anti-inflammatory that focuses on the lungs, so it can help reduce inflammation in the various passages and tissues in the lungs giving way to healing and easier breathing.

Mullein has been used traditionally as a tonic tea by people with asthma, COPD, emphysema, bronchitis, inflammation, respiratory allergies, recurring congestion, smoker's cough, exercise-induced lung strain, and anxiety-related breathing issues.

Mullein is calming, soothing, comforting, and very grounding. The tea on its own is actually very pleasant for those who like an 'earthy' taste in their tea. When combined with herbs that have stronger flavor profiles, the flavor of mullein will usually be lost.

Safety: As strong of a decongestant, irritation soother, and lung healer mullein is, it is equally gentle. Mullein is considered to be an extremely safe herb to take with no commonly known side effects or precautions.

Plantain
Plantago major
Leaves

Plantain has been my go-to cleansing herbs for years. I love the way it tastes, smells, and looks – and there's just something that strikes my intuition about this herb. I find it to be deeply comforting and reassuring, and I think you will too.

Plantain grows in places we humans might scoff at. Roadsides, abandoned parking lots, gutters, old buildings, and derelict yards. It pops up in places where it seems that cleansing, harmonizing, and a little TLC are most in need - and that applies equally to what it can do for our lungs.

One of the most problematic and uncomfortable things that can take place in the lungs is a buildup of phlegm and mucous in the lungs. No matter how deep, it seems we can always tell when just one passageway within our lungs isn't taking in air the way it should. In cases like this, plantain gets work helping to clear and remove these blockages so that we can breathe free once again. This is extremely important when the phlegm and mucous that are trapped have already taken a good deal of trapped toxins. We certainly don't want that stuff hanging around in our lungs any longer than it has to!

The mucous lining of the lungs is essential to their function. Healthy mucous traps toxins, debris, and pollutants before they get to the more vulnerable areas of our respiratory system. When mucous isn't healthy, none of the respiratory system can be healthy and we are open to a greater risk of illness. Plantain works hard to restore a healthier and stronger mucous lining throughout the lung and breathing tract which feels great!

Another blessing plantain brings to the all-important mucous lining is help in the area of inflammation, infection, and weakness. If there are small inflammatory cycles or even lingering infections in the lungs, plantain can help get them healed.

While you're enjoying the gentle and deep detox plantain gives your lungs, your entire body is also benefitting. Plantain helps cleanse and detoxify the blood so that it works better with the lungs and with all the other organs and functions of the body.

Safety: Plantain is considered to be extremely safe and gentle. There are no commonly known side effects or precautions. Do not use plantain if you are pregnant or breastfeeding without consulting a medical professional first.

Hyssop
Hyssopus officinalis
Stems, leaves, and flowers

Hyssop is famed for its ability to target the entire respiratory system and get things cleaned and strengthened at the same time. For many herbalists, hyssop is the go-to herb for people who deal with a wide array of respiratory diseases like asthma, chronic bronchitis, severe allergies, and emphysema.

Hyssop goes to work by first cleansing phlegm and mucous from the lungs – especially that which is filled with toxins or other particles. This plant is one of the most effective yet gentle expectorants, so when you use it you can expect to move a lot of gunk from your lungs! Once the phlegm and mucous has been cleansed, the anti-inflammatory effects of hyssop become apparent. The entire respiratory system is soothed as inflammation is removed and the mucous lining is restored back to health.

The main benefit you'll get from working with hyssop in your lung detox is deep cleaning. This herb goes deep into the lungs, moves out anything that's congesting or blocking healthy breathing, and then helps your system to build new mucous lining in an inflammation-free environment.

I suggest adding small amounts of hyssop to your blends at first, then increasing as you become comfortable with its expectorant effects. I tend to enjoy hyssop when I'll be home for several hours so that coughing and moving things from my lungs doesn't cause embarrassment. It's really that powerful!

Safety: Hyssop is an extremely safe and gentle herb to use for most healthy adults. Because of its strong expectorant effects, it should not be used during acute respiratory attacks like those associated with asthma. It is best used as a supportive tea when attacks are not happening. Pregnant women should avoid hyssop since it can cause uterine contractions. Hyssop is not a good choice for children and should be excluded from blends they may enjoy. Adults with a history of seizures should stay away from hyssop.

Peppermint
Mentha piperita
Leaves and tops

Not everyone is a fan of peppermint, but this is an essential herb to cover for a few reasons. First, it's a great flavor enhancer for fans of mint. Second, it does some amazing things for the lungs. Third, it's an easy and affordable herb to use that has a variety of applications in everyday life, so it's a great herb to have on hand. If you aren't a peppermint fan, have no fear. You can either use such a small amount in your tea blends that you don't even taste it, or you can replace it with one of the other alternatives I'll share next.

Peppermint tea has a long history of use both socially and medicinally. Its distinct flavor sets it apart from other herbal tea blends, and it tastes great hot or iced. Just smelling a brewing cup of peppermint herbal tea can get the process of decongestion started thanks to the powerful essential oils it contains!

Peppermint added to your herbal tea lung detox brings flavor, fragrance, and feel good. This herb is packed with personality, and it helps soothe the body, melt away tension, relax the mind, and open the lungs.

Safety: There are no known warnings or hazards with drinking peppermint tea. It is traditionally used liberally throughout Europe and no common side effects or precautions are noted.

Mullein, plantain, hyssop, and peppermint. These four herbs cover the most essential functions of the lungs and help cleanse, clear, soothe, and heal in the gentlest yet most powerful way. As you read, these herbs are all extremely safe and can be used with confidence when it comes to brewing herbal tea. If you choose no other herbs to work with when healing your lungs, these are the best in my opinion.

These four herbs have been chosen because they work together in perfect synergy. Mullein reaches up with its tall, lanky stalk to harness air energy and get the lungs working well again. Grounded plantain stays low to the ground and finds peace in the Earth. It offers deep and thorough cleansing on many levels. Hyssop is an ancient evergreen bush that offers deep cleansing and great strengthening for the entire respiratory system. Playful peppermint brings joy, calm, and positive energy so that the process of healing can be enjoyable. Together, they create a blend that gets the job done well while nurturing body, mind, emotions, energy, and soul along the way.

In order to arm you and your lungs with even more healing options, I want to briefly share just a few more herbal tea possibilities with you. Feel free to try any of these herbs out, and use them every few weeks once your 7-day detox is over to continue the nourishing you give your lungs.

Yerba Mate
Ilex paraguayensis
Leaves

Mate is a popular coffee-like drink that is favored in South America. It is packed with energy and rivals the stimulating properties of strong coffee. Because of its general tonic and stimulant effects, it makes a good general bronchodilator that can help making breathing easier.

Safety: Yerba mate is no cap of green tea! This herb packs a powerful stimulant property that can make seasoned coffee drinkers get the jitters. Drink slowly until you learn more about how it works with your system.

Lobelia

Lobelia inflate
Above ground parts

Lobelia is a powerful herb that can help transform long-time cigarette addicts into happy ex-smokers. I spend a lot of time exploring lobelia in my book 'Quitting Smoking With Herbal Tea'.

It's interesting that lobelia can help us quit smoking and then help rebuild the damage we've done to our lungs. It seems as if this plant has a very distinct purpose that acts as a deep blessing to those of us who struggle with smoking addiction.

Lobelia has been traditionally used with great success to treat a wide variety of respiratory ailments from recurring bronchitis and inflammation to smoker's cough and asthma.

Safety: Lobelia should not be used by those who have successfully quit smoking as it can mimic the effects of nicotine and cause relapse. Lobelia should be taken in very small doses to avoid a variety of unpleasant symptoms that seem to mirror those of nicotine poisoning.

Licorice Root
Glycyrrhiza glabra
Root

Licorice root is one of my favorite herbs to add to any lung-focused blend for a two reasons. First, the sweet flavor makes even the most bitter tea taste like a real treat! Second, and most importantly, this amazing herb is both an expectorant and a demulcent. This means that it helps the lungs purge mucous and phlegm while also coating the delicate linings of the respiratory system with a soothing mucilage layer.

Licorice root can also help the respiratory system and the whole body recover from illness and get strong again. It's anti-inflammatory which means it can help soothe lungs that are healing from quitting smoking or environmental stresses, and it's antispasmodic which means it can help relax muscles and ease the process of breathing.

Safety: It is considered unsafe to use licorice root if you are pregnant or are breastfeeding. If you take any medications that focus on hormones, thyroid, blood pressure, or heart health you should consult with your healthcare professional before using this herb.

Chamomile

Matricaria recutita
Matricaria chamomile
Chamaemelum nobile
Anthemis nobilis
Flowers

I've chosen to include chamomile in this list for one reason – it is the king of calm. Many times there is an underlying anxiety or stress behind the inability to breathe properly. When we get stressed, our diaphragm becomes tight and knotted. When this happens, we breathe shallowly with our shoulders and ribs and our lungs are not able to cleanse properly. In no time we end up with mucous and phlegm buildup and lungs that are only being worked superficially.

Using chamomile is a blissful way to love yourself and take time each day to just relax, let go, and receive. This herb is gentle, calming, soothing, emotionally balancing, uplifting, pain relieving, and positive. The fragrance and taste are reminiscent of apples and earth.

Safety: If you have hay fever or other similar plant allergies, test a small bit of chamomile to ensure you don't react the same way. Some people are severely allergic to chamomile. Otherwise, this is a very safe, gentle, and effective herbal tea that can be used often.

In the next section we'll embark on the 7-Day lung detox. I'll show you how to create herbal tea blends, when to drink them, and what other steps you can take to make this the most healing and empowering week for your lungs.

THE 7-DAY LUNG DETOX

Let the healing begin! It's time to embark on your own 7-day lung detox to help your lungs clean, heal, and strengthen using the power of healing herbal tea. Although the detox focuses on using tea, I will be adding in some extra things you can do to supercharge just how effective and powerful your week will be. Feel free to exclude anything that doesn't work for you, but please do consider trying all of it!

Before we get to the 7-day program, let's cover a few of the essentials that will come up along the way.

Water

The lungs must have water to heal. The mucous and phlegm linings of the lungs, the tissues, the muscles, and the process of respiration all need water in order to be healthy. If you aren't getting enough water in your life, this is the week to make the change! You'll already be drinking more water thanks to your tea consumption, so keep it up by having a reusable water bottle on hand to sip all day long. The positive changes being truly hydrated will make in your life will astound you!

Movement

The lungs don't work entirely on muscle action. They also require movement in order to be stretched, expanded, and toned. Do your best to get out for a brisk walk every day, or do as much as you can within your own health limits. This may not be the right week to start an intensive exercise program, but adding in walks, stairs, and stretching can be a big help.

Breathing

In the next chapter I'll give you some simple yet powerful breathing exercises that you can do to cleanse, strengthen, and heal your lungs. Please try them all and use them as much as you can. Taking time to exercise your lungs and retrain yourself into a healthier way of breathing can literally change everything!

Food

Eating healthy food this week is a good idea. Stick to light, fresh, seasonal, and healthy as much as you can. Fruits and vegetables have tons of nutrients and water, so they make a great option for healing your lungs. Staying away from dairy, meat, and wheat can give your body a chance to end inflammation cycles and clear out any toxins that may have built up.

Herbal Tea

Your herbal tea blends will be at the center of your detox. The process of selecting the herbs you chose, brewing them, and drinking them is both a meditation and a proactive move towards your greater health. Allow yourself to be empowered and cheered on by the tea – it's here to help!

Although the detox is set up to last for 7 days, you can adjust it as needed or as suggested by your health care practitioner. A 3-day, 5-day, or even 9-day lung detox is fine as long as it works for your unique needs. I wouldn't suggest focusing on a detox for longer than 9 days.

Each of the 7 days will have some basic reminders of things to do that day. Again, take what is healthy, safe, or appropriate for you and leave the rest. You can always do a gentle detox for 3 days and come back a few months later for a more intense 7-day run once you know the process.

DAY ONE

Today is tea day! Brew your first cup of lung detox tea (see recipes section). Take time to look at the herbs you chose, get accustomed to their color and shape, smell them, and really just connect to them. The more you do this the more relaxed your body and mind will be about allowing them to do their work.

You may start with just one cup today, or drink up to three cups over the course of the whole day. Give about 3-4 hours between cups to see how the tea works with your body.

DAY TWO

If you only did one cup yesterday, bring yourself up to two or three cups today. If you started with two or three cups yesterday, continue that pace today.

DAY THREE

Drink two to three cups of your tea over the course of the whole day.

Participate in some type of movement like walking, taking stairs, or stretching in order to help your lungs cleanse and heal.

Drink water!

DAY FOUR

Drink two to three cups of your tea over the course of the whole day.

Participate in some type of movement like walking, taking stairs, or stretching in order to help your lungs cleanse and heal.

Do 3 to 5 minutes of a breathing exercise of your choice. See the next chapter for simple instructions.

Drink water!

DAY FIVE

Drink two to three cups of your tea over the course of the whole day.

Participate in some type of movement like walking, taking stairs, or stretching in order to help your lungs cleanse and heal.

Do two sets of 3 to 5 minutes of a breathing exercise of your choice with 6 to 8 hours between them. See the next chapter for simple instructions.

Drink water!

DAY SIX

Drink two to three cups of your tea over the course of the whole day.

Participate in some type of movement like walking, taking stairs, or stretching in order to help your lungs cleanse and heal.

Do two sets of 3 to 5 minutes of a breathing exercise of your choice with 6 to 8 hours between them. See the next chapter for simple instructions.

Drink water!

DAY SEVEN

Can you believe the week is already over?

Drink two to three cups of your tea over the course of the whole day.

Participate in some type of movement like walking, taking stairs, or stretching in order to help your lungs cleanse and heal.

Do two sets of 3 to 5 minutes of a breathing exercise of your choice with 6 to 8 hours between them. See the next chapter for simple instructions.

Drink water!

Congratulations!

You just spent 7 days loving your lungs and giving them the support, nourishment, and attention that can help them make drastic changes in just how healthy and strong they are.

Feel free to repeat your detox every 4-6 months as needed, and feel free to drink a cup of your lung tea whenever you feel like your lungs may need a little extra TLC. If you worked with the breathing exercises, keep it up! The more you practice the better your body will be at breathing in the best way possible. Soon it will become second nature and a completely effortless process that will happen for you all the time!

I the next chapter I'll be showing you some simple breathing exercises that will help retrain your body into the best way to breathe for overall health while helping your lungs to cleanse and clear. I'll also teach you a simple meditation that will help you draw in healing energy to your lungs as an act of gratitude and self-care whenever you need it.

EMPOWERING LUNG EXERCISES

In the modern day very few of us know how to breathe properly. As mentioned earlier, healthy breathing is good for the lungs, the organs, the processes of the body, our stress and immunity, and the world around us. If you discovered that your breathing isn't really up to par, these exercises will help you retrain your body back to a gentle, deep, and powerful breathing pattern.

If you have any concerns about engaging in breathing exercises, please consult your health care practitioner. If you experience discomfort or pain while doing these exercises, take a break and consider meeting with a respiratory therapist for some great one-on-one guidance in these and other techniques.

Harmonizing Cycles

In this simple exercise we're going to help cool the respiratory system and bring it into a state of balance. You can sit or stand for this practice, and after you've read the instructions a few times you can even do it while you're on the go. This may seem simple, but it's actually very refreshing, calming, and empowering for the lungs, mind, emotions, and body.

- Bring your attention to the tip of your nose and try to feel the air pass it as you inhale gently. Just try to experience the place where air enters your body.

- When it's time to exhale, bring your attention to your mouth and feel the air escaping gently through lightly pursed lips.
- Don't change or force the pattern of your breathing. Instead, just be there for it and try to watch it rise and fall, open and close, expand and contract. Get in touch with the beautiful rhythm of your breathing.
- Once you feel connected, try to follow your breath all the way from your nose to your belly and back out through your mouth. Imagine, pretend, or visualize the breath entering, going deep within, and then exiting. Try to go along for the ride.

This exercise helps regulate the flow of breath, helps generate awareness and gratitude for the process of breathing, and helps relax the mind. All good things!

Belly Breathing

The best and most healing way to breathe is with the belly. This exercise will allow you to spend a few minutes aligning your breathing to your belly so that your body can breathe deep, gentle, and powerful.

You can either lie on your back or sit in a flat-backed chair for this exercise. After you've done it a few times you can even do it while engaged in other activities!

- Take a few natural breaths and pay attention to which parts of your body move. Notice if you're

43

breathing with your shoulders, ribs, back, diaphragm, or belly.

- Place a hand on the area just below your navel. Try to connect with this area and feel is from within.
- Begin gently and without force guiding the area under your hand to effortlessly move out when you inhale and sink in when you exhale. Try to feel that when the belly moves out, air is naturally pulled into the lungs instead of being forced into the lungs when other muscle groups are involved.
- Try to breathe in through your nose, and out through gently pursed lips.
- Do not consider the look of your belly. It will pop out. Embrace it! This is not a time to worry about your silhouette or waist line. Let go completely and give your body a break from the holding and sucking in for a few minutes.
- Try to continue this exercise until your breathe is pulled in by the diaphragm muscle and belly, and until you feel as though your breath moves all the way down into your belly region. Practice makes perfect, so don't get upset if your body resists a bit the first few times. If you've been an unhealthy breather for a long time, this may be a process that you have to spend time, patience, and gentleness working on.

Cleansing Breathwork

In this exercise we will be using creative meditation and visualization to help the lungs clear and cleanse. You don't have to have any meditation or visualization experience at all to make this work for you. Just have fun with it and be willing to practice.

- You may sit or stand for this exercise, but it's best to be in a completely relaxed state. Try to position your body so that you can really let go and surrender to the floor or chair you're in. Take a moment to get really comfortable and adjust your body as needed.
- Just like we did in the *harmonizing cycles* exercise, start to watch and follow your breath. Get in touch with the flow and adjust yourself to make it as effortless and gentle as possible.
- When you are really experiencing the process of inhaling and exhaling, you can start the cleansing visualization.
- As you inhale, imagine clean, healing, pure, empowering air coming into your body. You may pretend this looks like light, imagine it as a cloud of healing energy, or sense it as a mist of nature's medicine. Do what works for you and take as many inhalations as you need to really connect to what works. You can see it in your mind's eye, sense it, or do anything else that connects you.
- When the healing air comes into your body and your inhalation draws to a finish, sense it being absorbed and accepted. In just an instant try to

45

imagine the good energy and healing of the breath being received by your entire being. Don't hold your breath to do this. Work yourself into a place where you can experience a 'flash' of acceptance as soon as it's time to end the inhalation.

- On the exhalation, imagine, visualize, pretend, or sense that any gunk, illness, imbalance, or stagnation is swept out of your lungs with the breath. You may see this as a gray cloud of smoke (excellent for smokers and ex-smokers), sense it as a sticky heaviness, or imagine it as dirty air. Try to experience your lungs openly releasing and expelling anything that isn't in their highest good.
- At the end of the exhalation, know that the toxins you expelled will be instantly healed and neutralized by the light of the sun, the earth, the clean air around you, or anything else that works in the moment. You will not be re-absorbing any of this and you won't send it out for anyone else to take in either.
- Continue breathing in healing and cleansing and breathing out toxins, dirt, weakness, and imbalance. Do this until you feel as though your lungs are telling you to stop, or until you notice that your exhalation visualizations become less and less dirty and eventually pure like the air you breathe in.

This is a wonderful exercise to do first thing in the morning, as you lay in bed at night, just before or after exercise, or while you're waiting for your herbal tea to steep.

The three simple exercises shared above help open the lungs, deepen the breathing, activate the diaphragm, relieve stress and tension within the respiratory process, remove toxins, and connect you to your sacred breath. They may seem simple, but these techniques have been used in many forms of alternative healing for centuries and in the modern day by many respiratory therapists as well.

Your lungs are an integral and living part f your body. The more you care for them, strengthen them, and even listen to them – the healthier they will be! Working with the healing power of herbal tea while taking proactive steps to love your lungs is a true life changer. As your lungs heal and strengthen, you may just find that other parts of your body, mind, emotions, and life do the same.

Here's to the power of breath!

LUNG LOVING HERBAL TEA RECIPES

Here are a few of my personal favorite herbal tea blends that love the lungs!

Essential Lung Detox Blend
Use this recipe for your daily detox tea

½ t. Mullein
½ t. Plantain
A pinch of Licorice Root (optional)
A pinch to ¼ t. of Hyssop (optional)
Pinch of Peppermint or Chamomile

Steep 6 minutes in 8oz. just-boiling water.

Deep Cleanse Blend

½ t. Plantain
½ t. Hyssop
Pinch of Chamomile

Steep 6 minutes in 8oz. just-boiling water.

This is a systemic detox blend with a focus on the lungs. It's best before bed after a day of great hydration so that your body can cleanse while you rest.

StimuLung

½ t. Yerba Mate
½ t. Mullein

Steep 6 minutes in 8oz. just-boiling water.

This is a highly stimulant tea that opens the lungs and can make breathing easier. Yerba Mate is best avoided by people who don't like intense caffeine-like stimulants.

Happy Lungs Iced Herbal Tea

1 t. Peppermint
1 t. Mullein
½ t. Chamomile
A pinch of Licorice Root

This tea is made strong since it will be watered down with ice. If you won't be using ice, cut back the quantities by about 25%.

Add herbs to a lidded glass jar like a canning jar. Top off with about 10 ounces of clean water. Place in the refrigerator for 4-6 hours. Separate tea from water by using a sieve, strainer, or mesh infuser bowl. Add ice and enjoy!

Breathe Joyful - Fresh Fruit Herbal Tea

½ Orange (or your choice of citrus fruit)
¼ Lemon or Lime
5-6 Berries, your choice
1 t. Peppermint
½ t. Ginger Root
½ t. Chamomile
½ t. Mullein

Slice up the fruit thinly. Crush the berries. Add fruit slices, berries, and dried herbs to a lidded glass jar, and then top off with about 10 ounces of clean water. Refrigerate for 4-6 hours, separate herbs and fruits from water with a strainer, add ice if desired, and enjoy!

REFERENCES

McKeown, Patrick. *Close Your Mouth.* Asthma Care Publishing, 2004.

Cohen, Ken. *The Way Of Qigong.* Wellspring/Ballantine, 1999.

Cohen, Ken. *Taoist Breathing.* Sounds True, 2012

Zak, Victoria. *20,000 Secrets Of Tea.* Dell Publishing, 1999.

Antol, Marie Nadine. *Healing Teas.* Avery Trade, 1995.

Ritchason, Jack, N.D. *The Little Herb Encyclopedia.* Woodland Health Books, 1995

Blumenthal, Mark. *The ABC Clinical Guide To Herbs.* American Botanical Council, 2003.

www.WebMD.com

ABOUT THE AUTHOR

Josh Williams is an herbal tea healing enthusiast who lives in the Mountain West. He works to introduce people to the healing and empowering potentials of plant medicine through herbal tea, and love educating, sharing, and creating new healing tea recipes.

Josh can be found online at

www.LivingHerbalTea.com

Other books by Josh Williams...

Quit Smoking With Herbal Tea

Healing Herbal Tea For Stress, Worry, and Anxiety

Herbal Tea 101